Strandtastic

VOLUME 1

A Guide to Growing Healthy Natural Hair

Strandtastic

VOLUME 1

A Guide to Growing Healthy Natural Hair

ZAKIYA ANTOINE, DO, MPH

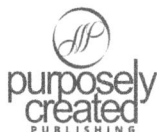

purposely
created
PUBLISHING

STRANDTASTIC VOLUME I
Published by Purposely Created Publishing Group™

Copyright © 2019 Zakiya Antoine

Printed in the United States of America

ISBN: 978-1-64484-016-0

Special discounts are available on bulk quantity purchases by book clubs, associations and special interest groups. For details email: sales@publishyourgift.com or call (888) 949-6228.

For information log on to www.PublishYourGift.com

Table of Contents

Acknowledgments

To the natural hair and makeup community on social media, especially on YouTube,

You guys not only indirectly inspired this book, but you saved me from a very dark time in my life when I didn't like myself. I had let life beat me down so much while I was in medical school that I neglected my appearance, my health, and my hair. I did not know it at the time, but I was clinically depressed. Through working on my outward physical appearance, I began to heal on the inside. Somehow this community helped put me back together piece by piece until I was whole again. If you are a beauty influencer on YouTube, I love you—even if we have never met. You may not realize it, but you help transform people's lives. I know this because you helped transform mine. I went from a depressed, damaged-hair diva with little to no makeup skills to a confident, "born-again" beauty junkie who would never let her passive aggressive antagonists at her internship, residency, or moonlighting jobs get the best of her. For this reason, I deeply and humbly thank *all* of you.

To my mom and dad,
Thank you for your unwavering support through every phase of my life from birth to this very moment, as I publish my

book based on my passions and purpose here on Earth. Thank you for believing in me and giving me the tools I need to succeed in life. You have always instilled in me that I can achieve any goal I set for myself. From teaching me how to read at three years old to buying my first chemistry set at eleven years old because I was fascinated with science, you guys have never wavered in your love and support. For this reason, I know I am so blessed to have the two of you as my parents. I love you both unconditionally. I owe everything I am to both of you for loving me and supporting me always.

To my late cousin, Brandon Allen Small,

Thank you for all those late night talks about life, love, medicine, money, and entrepreneurship. I can't believe you won't get to read this book because this book signifies the start of the part of my life we always envisioned. I know that you helped me write this book because I thought about you every day while writing it. I will always miss those random, funny stories you would call to tell me in the middle of the night while I was home for a visit that would make me laugh so hard I would wake my parents with our banter. Thank you for always supporting me, cuz. I love you.

To my business coach, dear friend, and mentor, Dr. Draion Burch,

I'm so glad that I didn't listen when "they" told me to "consider the source" after "they" found out you were helping me adjust to life as a young woman who had just found out that she was accepted to medical school. The dynamic transformation that I have made from medical student to Medical Mogul is all because of you. Although you may not fess up to it, you were my coach well before you were even thinking about charging me for any of your coaching programs. Thank you for always pushing me to aspire to greatness. You do not know how many times you have saved me from myself and from the malignant culture we both endured as young minority medical students and residents. This book would not even be in existence if not for your connections, vision, and foresight. Thank you for your encouragement, support, and most of all, your friendship. I love you and appreciate how you have always been that person cheering me on and watching me from the sidelines since that fateful day we met in Athens, Ohio.

Foreword

The natural hair care industry has been on a steady incline for many years now, but it holds true that women of color and their special hair needs remain an underserved entity in the United States today. More women are going "natural" or using organic hair products in their hair. When I first began a journey to embrace my natural coils/curls ten years ago, I found myself discouraged by the lack of products out there that would help my hair thrive. In fact, I was so discouraged that I was motivated enough to take action to create my own natural hair brand to create hair products that were natural and safe. Today, there is an ever-growing number of brands for consumers with naturally curly/coil hair. In the past, it was more common to leave department stores without products that were created for multi-cultural hair. Now, women need help navigating through this section of the store to decide which products will give the desired effect or which products are appropriate for their hair type. Although the number of suitable products in the market have grown, many women still yearn for the knowledge to empower themselves in caring for their hair, purchasing safe hair products, and growing healthy, longer hair.

I had the pleasure of meeting Dr. Zakiya through common business associates after she was present for a live social media event for beauty business entrepreneurs where I was a guest speaker. She approached me and suggested that I write the foreword for her upcoming book because she was inspired by my comments about the reason why I got started in the hair care industry years ago. Motivated to embrace her own natural hair after years of relaxers, Dr. Zakiya began to notice her black female patients were spending more time asking her about her hair regimen for themselves or their children instead of focusing on the reason for their visit to the urgent care clinic where she was working. She told me that is when she realized how important hair is to women, and she also realized that there was a great need for the general public to be properly informed on how to care for their natural hair. I was humbled at the thought of her wanting me to be a part of her project, and I think her science background and extensive training in medicine give her more than enough credibility as an expert on this topic.

Trust me when I say this is not your average "how to" book. Writing for her followers who she affectionately calls #Curlfriends, Dr. Zakiya shares her personal hair struggles and stories using her fun voice. As you read this book, try to think of ways to incorporate the knowledge that Dr. Zakiya is sharing with you to help retain more length, transition your relaxed hair to natural, and care properly for your own hair while using protective styles. This book offers the basic fundamentals of naturally curly hair and offers insight on ways to help your hair flourish. As you take this natural hair journey, using the pointers Dr. Zakiya provides, you will be ultimately empowered to begin the transition to make your hair, StrandTASTIC!

Pamela J. Booker
Founder/CEO of Koils By Nature

A Note to the Reader

Hi #Curlfriends! If you have purchased this book, then you either have seen me on social media discussing natural hair or have a desire to learn more about natural hair and how to care for it properly to stimulate and support growth and length retention. I once was in the same position you are in at this very moment. There are many resources out there, but I was always on the hunt for more knowledge that was concise, easy to understand, and fun to read. For years, I combed through Internet blogs, YouTube tutorials, and hair magazines, trying to satisfy my quest for the natural hair knowledge I yearned to have. So, if your quest for knowledge has led you to purchasing my book, I humbly thank you. You could have purchased any other resource out there, but you didn't. You chose to rock with your girl! For this reason, I truly appreciate you! I have tried to make this piece of literature as concise and complete as possible, but you also get Dr. Zakiya's fun personality and spin on some of the same topics you have been coming across in your research. You will find a recurrent theme in this book that focuses on maintaining a balance between moisture and protein along with other nutrients to help restore and refresh your natural hair in order to promote length retention. So without any further adieu, let's get this party started.

My Story

Hi! I am Dr. Zakiya, board-certified family medicine physician and natural hair expert. I have excelled academically all my life. I was introduced to medicine when I was only eight years old through my experiences in the Girl Scouts of the USA. From the moment I decided to become a doctor, I became determined to put forth the extra effort required to get ahead in life. I made straight As and won every award that a young girl could win in elementary school. One year, I received so many awards at our annual Spring Award Ceremony that I could not hold them all in my tiny, nine-year-old arms. My mom was so proud—she had taken the afternoon off from her job to be there to see her baby girl receive all her awards.

This was a normal occurrence for me from elementary school through high school, where I finished as an honor graduate at the top of my class with a full scholarship to Xavier University of Louisiana to become a pre-med major. At Xavier, I continued to excel. I made the Dean's List and received more scholarship money. I even had a 4.0 for a few semesters. I was invited to join academic honor societies that were only for students who had high GPAs in the sciences. After again graduating with distinction from college, I continued my education at Tulane University where I obtained my master of public health before continuing on to Ohio University to complete my doctorate in osteopathic medicine. During my first two years of medical school, I again excelled academically and was at the top of my class.

My story sounds pretty awesome up to this point, doesn't it? Who wouldn't want to have an educational foundation that sets you on the path to what most assume will be a successful career and happy life? But, I had a secret.

By the time I was set to graduate medical school, I was not happy. It was not because I was failing, and it was not because I couldn't rise to meet the demands of the busy schedule of a fourth-year medical student. I was unhappy because although I had achieved my goal of becoming a physician, my life was nothing like the dream I had as an eight-year-old girl. I had envisioned myself to be ecstatic at the thought of achieving my childhood dream. I imagined I would have fulfilling relationships with the attending physicians who were in charge of training me. I thought that these established physicians would be morally ethical and would exhibit supportive behavior toward me. I thought that the person who had been my best friend for the last four years would be standing next to me on graduation day with a stupid grin on his face because he too was excited about our blossoming careers as resident physicians.

Instead, my reality was that I was stretched to the limit in my personal life due to the malignant practices at the hospital where I trained. There were preceptors who lied about my performance on my medical rotations and gossiped about me like teenagers, instead of acting like the professionals they were supposed to be. The same preceptors had me doing their research and PowerPoint presentations and put their own name on them as if they worked on them with me—but they hadn't!

The last straw was when one of the few medical students in my class, the one I considered to be my best friend and a trusted source of support during this turmoil, chose to perform a betrayal so devious and hurtful that I had no choice but to end our four-year friendship. This so-called best friend, who I had confided in for years, chose this time to act like I was aggressively "stalking him" to make himself look better to a girl he was dating who was secretly jealous of our friendship. I felt especially betrayed because he had also displayed other toxic behavior toward me.

As a result, I started neglecting myself and became very withdrawn. When I finally went home to prepare for graduation, I had unintentionally dropped thirty pounds, and much of my hair was thinning and falling out. I was so devastated that I did not even want to attend my medical school graduation.

Because of these experiences, I ultimately was influenced to start a beauty brand that could help all women transform their self-image, enhance their natural beauty, and regain their self-confidence. When women feel their outward appearance is at its best, they feel better about themselves and create more opportunities for themselves. Now I want all of you to live your best lives and know that you will look *amazing* while doing so!

Basic Hair Anatomy

What would a self-help book written by a medical doctor be without science? I have to start off with the basics so you guys can understand why natural hair products are created to help women of color solve a specific set of problems with their hair. I promise—I will not take the fun out of it.

Your hair strands have two basic components: the **hair follicle** and the **hair shaft**. The **hair follicle** is considered to be the "living portion" of your hair because it has a blood supply and contains living cells that are influenced by hormones that stimulate hair growth.

The hair follicle consists of the:

- **papilla** – structure located at the base of the hair follicle that contains capillaries and connective tissue

- **root sheath** – comprised of an external root sheath and an internal root sheath; basically contains cells and an internal layer that connects with the outermost portion of your cuticle

Other noteworthy structures that reside in the hair follicle are the arrector pilli muscle and sebaceous glands. The **arrector pilli muscle** is responsible for causing the hair follicle to become more perpendicular to the skin and protrude above its surrounding skin, a.k.a. goosebumps. **Sebaceous glands** are oil-producing glands that produce sebum or a waxy substance that coats the hair. As the hair becomes denser, the number of follicles increases, with a direct proportion of the increase in sebaceous glands.

The **hair shaft** is considered to be the "dead portion" of your hair because it is made up of three separate layers of keratin or protein:

- **inner layer (medulla)**
- **middle layer (cortex)** – contains pigments for hair color
- **outer layer (cuticle)** – stacked like shingles, one on top of the other throughout hair shaft

The cuticle is the hair shaft's protective layer that is the point of focus for most products that are created to condition the hair. These products condition the hair by "smoothing out" the cuticle.

HAIR ANATOMY

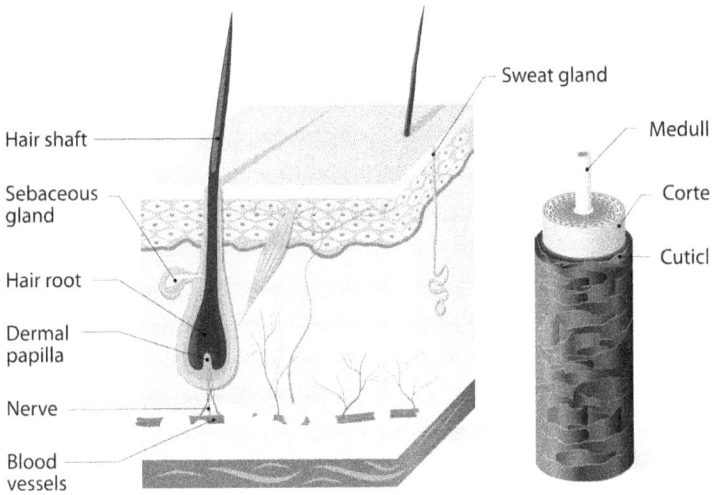

Hair shaft

Sebaceous gland

Hair root

Dermal papilla

Nerve

Blood vessels

Sweat gland

Medull

Corte

Cuticl

Notes

Notes

_____

_____

_____

_____

_____

_____

_____

_____

_____

_____

_____

_____

_____

_____

_____

_____

_____

_____

_____

Notes

Notes

Hair Physiology, a.k.a. the Growth Cycle

Understanding the basic physiology of your hair's growth cycle can shed some light on why some of you may not have been able to grow your hair past a certain length. As hard as it may be for some of you to believe, our hair is growing at a rate of at least 1mm per day. That is a rate of at least 6 inches per year. If your hair is not showing noticeable signs of growth, then you are not retaining length.

Length retention is a completely different phenomenon from hair growth. Length retention is a process that entails retaining the length on the ends of the hair. The ends are the oldest part of your hair and also the most fragile. This means to really see noticeable signs of hair growth, you must protect the ends of your hair to retain the growth that occurs at the level of the scalp. Hair growth and hair loss are not seasonal or cyclical. Hair growth is a random process that causes our strands to be in various stages of growth or shedding at any given time. There are three phases of the growth cycle:

1. **Anagen Phase:** This is the growth phase of your hair strands. Most of your strands are constantly growing in

this phase. Hair strands can remain in this phase for up to four years. Some of you may be having trouble with hair growth because you have a short anagen phase. Those of you with long hair most likely have a long anagen phase.

2. **Catagen Phase:** This is a transitional phase that contains about 3 percent of the total number of your hair strands. During this transitional phase, which can last from one to two weeks, hair growth slows down. After the process is complete, your strands have become **club hairs** that will eventually become hairs that you will shed. Club hairs are named as such because of the solid, white material found at the root if you pull one of these hairs from your head. It is normal to shed about 100 hairs per day.

3. **Telogen Phase:** This is a resting phase that can last up to four months until you finally shed your club hairs from the catagen phase.

Human hair growth

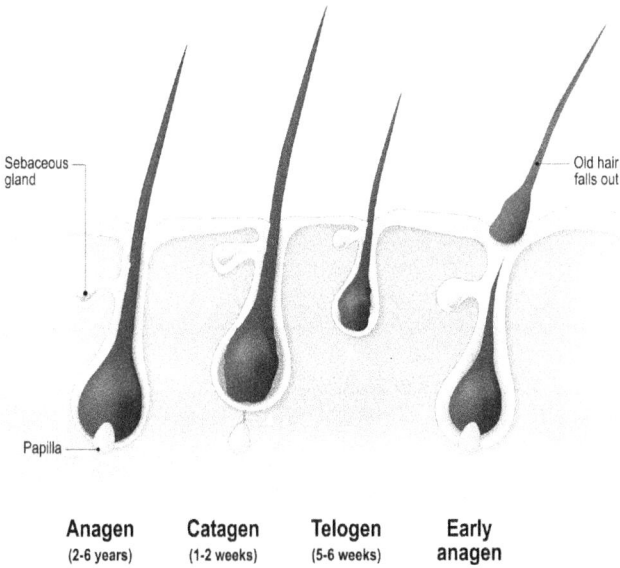

Sebaceous gland

Old hair falls out

Papilla

Anagen	Catagen	Telogen	Early anagen
(2-6 years)	(1-2 weeks)	(5-6 weeks)	

Notes

Notes

_____

_____

_____

_____

_____

_____

_____

_____

_____

_____

_____

_____

_____

_____

_____

_____

_____

_____

Notes

Notes

So, you guys should probably take notes on this section. If you can truly understand this information and apply it to your own hair to determine your true hair type, you will be ahead of the game when heading to your local department or beauty supply store to pick up natural hair products to nurture and style your hair. To start, I will go over the **four hair types** and their classification system, which was created by a man named Andre Walker, who is well known as Oprah Winfrey's hair stylist. This is the most common hair typing system mentioned in social media literature that refers to **curl pattern**. Please look at the picture of the Andre Walker Classification System below:

HAIR TYPE

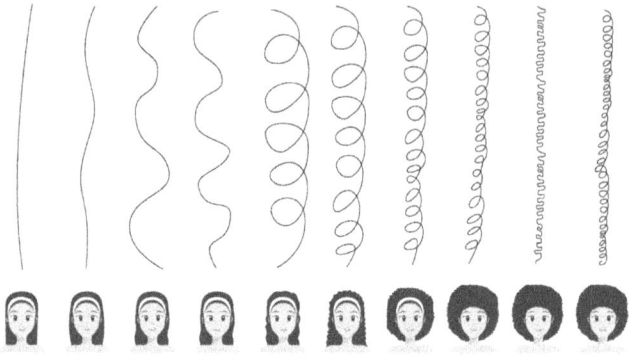

As you all can see now, **type 1** hair is completely straight, and **type 2** hair is slightly wavy. **Type 3** hair is curly, and **type 4** hair is very tight curls or coils.

Type 3 and type 4 hair are further divided into three subgroups that are represented by the letters *a*, *b*, and *c*. These letters refer to the diameter of your curls. Type a curls represent the biggest and looser curls, while type c curls are the smallest and tighter curls. This information is useful when choosing how to style your hair, but it does not help with deciding what methods to use to moisturize the hair. This chart also supports the controversial "good" versus "bad" hair comments that a lot of people make when talking about certain hair textures. We all can have "good" hair if we know our hair's characteristics. The Andre Walker system only accounts for the way your hair looks as it grows out of the scalp. It does not account for the texture or how it feels as you manipulate the hair with your hands. Neither does it account for the amount of hair strands that a person may have on his or her head. Finally, it does not account for the way your strands will absorb, retain moisture, or respond to stretching. All of these characteristics play a role in a routine that you should develop to manage and care for your natural hair.

Hair texture can be fine, normal/medium, or coarse/thick. Hair texture is a direct correlation to the diameter of your hair shaft. **Fine hair** is very delicate and prone to breakage if it is not moisturized adequately because it has less of a protein structure than any other texture. Fine hair does not hold curls well and tends to be very frizzy. **Normal hair** texture is not as delicate as fine hair because it has more protein in its structure. **Normal/medium texture** holds curls better than fine hair. It tends to be more pliable as well. **Coarse/thick hair** holds curls the best, but it is not as pliable as its fine or medium counterparts. Is it possible to have different textures and curl patterns in one head of hair? Yes! If we didn't have enough trouble understanding the type of curls and the texture of our hair, Mother Nature wanted to be sure we were confused by giving us multiple textures and curl patterns in one head of hair.

Hair density refers to the amount of strands on your head. People with high-density or thick hair have many strands of hair that are packed closely together in the scalp. Thin or low-density hair does not have as many strands packed closely together and can have issues with braids, twists, or clip-in extensions. You cannot put a lot of tension on low-density hair.

Hair porosity refers to the way your strands absorb and retain moisture. Normal-porosity hair has no problems with receiving or retaining moisture. High-porosity hair is very easily moisturized because the hair cuticle is open. The main disadvantage of high-porosity hair is that it loses moisture just as easily as it absorbs it. Sometimes high-porosity hair can be caused by chemical, heat, and mechanical damage to the hair cuticle. It can be a struggle to maintain appropriate moisture levels in damaged high-porosity hair. Low-porosity hair is characterized by strands that have a tightly closed cuticle, which makes it difficult to moisturize this type of hair. However, it looks great once moisturized. This is important information because naturally curly type 3 and type 4 hair love moisture. It's also important to know that **moisture is one of the necessities for length retention and hair health**.

You cannot get the appropriate amount of moisture in your strands if you cannot decipher the porosity of your hair. It is also important to note that heat, age, chemicals, and medications can change the porosity of your hair.

Hair elasticity refers to the ability of your hair to be stretched and then return to its normal state. Healthy hair should be able to be stretched at least 50 percent or more and return to its normal state after wetting it. Unhealthy hair will not be able to be stretched past 15 to 20 percent. Inelastic hair is more prone to breakage and damage with heavy manipulation styling, especially heat styling tools or rollers.

*Fun Fact: Dr. Zakiya has fine, dense, normal- to high-porosity, type 3b-3c curls.

Notes

Notes

Notes

Notes

Hair Maintenance

Okay—there is a lot of talk about how often us curly girls should be washing, conditioning, and trimming our hair. My secret is that I only shampoo once or sometimes twice per month. My best advice to all of you reading this book is to evaluate your current regimen after reading my book to see if there are some changes that you may need to make to your current regimen (if you have one). My basic requirements for type 3 or type 4 hair maintenance include the regular use of shampoo and co-washes. Now—I already know that some of you do not know what I am talking about when I bring up the word "co-wash." Well, sis, I am about to tell you.

A **co-wash** is a conditioner that is used to cleanse the hair. Most times, co-washing consists of using a moisturizing conditioner on your wet hair (instead of a shampoo); then just simply comb it through before rinsing it out of your hair. There are some co-washes that have gentle cleansing agents to help remove the buildup of dirt and other impurities from your scalp, which I review in depth in a later chapter of this book. You guys should definitely be using shampoo once every two weeks at minimum. If you need to cleanse or refresh your hair more frequently without stripping it of moisture, then you should consider using a co-wash in between shampoo sessions. Now, do not co-wash your hair every day just because you think it's something neutral. I have seen many naturalistas prevent themselves from retaining length by cleansing their hair and scalp too much. Their scalp became irritated and inflamed from the overuse of these products. So I approve using shampoo once per week or once every other week while using a co-wash or conditioner to freshen your hair without stripping it of the necessary moisture. Moisture is an important part of maintaining healthy, natural hair and retaining length.

If you must shampoo your hair every week because you work out often or just have oily hair, then I recommend you pre-poo your hair first. What is a pre-poo? A **pre-poo** consists of applying a moisturizing treatment to the hair prior to applying shampoo to cleanse the hair. A pre-poo can be a cheap rinse-out conditioner, coconut oil, or olive oil. Most naturalistas divide their hair into four sections, apply their pre-poo treatment, and then finally cover their hair with a plastic cap sometimes leaving it in overnight. This is a great idea for people who have lots of thick curly hair that tends to get tangled on wash day.

Another great maintenance tip is to trim all your split ends. I have quizzed many naturalistas who have waist-length hair. They have all told me that they only trim their hair one to two times per year. You must use the proper tools to trim your hair, i.e., hair shears—not paper scissors. Please do not cut your hair with the dull pair of paper scissors that you have had lying around your house for the last few years. This will produce counterproductive results if you are trying to grow your hair past your bra strap like me. These scissors are not sharp enough. When using dull scissors to cut your hair, you do not remove the split ends but instead cause the damaged ends of your hair to remain present, which prevents the length retention that you are aiming to achieve.

Finally, find deep conditioners that help you restore the moisture–protein balance to your hair. I deep condition my hair two times per week. Most times, I am using a moisturizing deep conditioner. However, I also recommend using a deep conditioner with protein in it at least one to two times per month, depending on your hair porosity and hair type.

Notes

Notes

Notes

Notes

_____

_____

_____

_____

_____

_____

_____

_____

_____

_____

_____

_____

_____

_____

_____

_____

_____

_____

Common Hair and Scalp Disorders

Throughout my years of medical training, I have seen many different problems that arise in the hair and scalp. I'd like to talk about some of the most common ailments at this time because I know you guys want to know about these disorders. I'm sure that most of you have seen these too, although you may not be familiar with the correct medical terms.

Trichodystrophy: Defective nutrition or growth of hair that often results in alopecia. This disease can be acquired or congenital.

Folliculitis: This word translates from its Latin derivatives (*folliculus* + *itis*) as inflammation of the follicle. This inflammation is usually caused by an infection with an organism by the name of *Staphylococcus aureus*. It is treated with antibiotics. This disease process is not limited to only the scalp, and it can occur in any area of your body that has hair.

Dandruff (Seborrheic Dermatitis): Who hasn't had a dry, flaky scalp at one time or another? This disease process is characterized by continuous inflammation of the scalp accompanied by dryness, itchiness, and flaky dead skin. People with excessive itchiness and flakiness often need treatment with prescription-strength anti-fungal shampoo or anti-dandruff shampoo.

Head Lice (Pediculosis Capitis): I know some of you may have had issues with this common infestation. The louse is a tiny insect that infests the human scalp and feeds on your blood supply in the scalp. It reproduces by laying tiny white eggs in your hair. It is most common in elementary- and middle-school-aged children and the adults who live with them, as this infestation is spread through close contact with carriers.

Ringworm (Tinea Capitis): Tinea is a common fungal infection that occurs in the scalp and is often named by the location of the body that it infects. Ringworm is another disease process that can invade many different locations of the human body. So please do not be confused by this fancy medical term that indicates that this infection is in the scalp.

Piedra (Trichomycosis Nodularis): This disease process is characterized by a fungal infection of the hair shaft (not the scalp). This disease consists of hard nodules of fungus that cling to the hair strands and can lead to hair loss.

Aloepecia Areata: Hair loss that is characterized by round patches of total hair loss from the scalp. The cause is unknown, but the hair usually grows back. Thank God!

Traction Alopecia: This is one of the most common causes of hair loss in African American women who wear weaves and braided hairstyles due to the tension force being applied to the hair. It can lead to scarring of the scalp.

Central Centrifugal Cicatrical Alopecia (CCCA): This is another common cause of hair loss in African American females. It normally starts as a gradual process at the crown of the scalp and spreads in a circular or centrifugal pattern. CCCA causes destruction of the hair follicle and leads to scarring that causes permanent hair loss. It is believed that is caused by excessive use of harsh chemicals in relaxers, braided hairstyles, hot combs, and excessive heat and hot oils on the scalp. It is best to seek treatment for this disease before permanent scarring and subsequent permanent hair loss results. Common methods to treat this disease are oral, topical, or injected corticosteroids, oral antibiotics, and other anti-inflammatory agents to reduce scalp inflammation and hair loss. I spent two months with a dermatologist during my training as a family medicine resident. I saw so many black women come in to get injections in their scalp to treat CCCA. I was so glad that I had stopped using relaxers at that point, but I was still wearing sew-in extensions. I finally started to contemplate the damage I was doing to my own hair.

Telogen Effluvium: Hair loss that occurs a month or two after a personal traumatic shock (surgery, severe stress, or depression). No treatment is necessary as hair usually starts growing back right away.

Anagen Effluvium: This is a longer-term type and often includes thinning or loss of other body hair, including eyebrows and eyelashes. Anagen effluvium takes place during the hair's "new growth" phase.

Postpartum Alopecia: Hair loss that occurs after delivering a baby; this is a specific subtype of telogen effluvium and usually resolves on its own. The exact cause is unknown.

Hirsutism: A condition characterized by the growth of male pattern hair on a women (i.e., facial hair) that is usually caused by excess testosterone production. Women seeking to get this hair permanently removed usually get laser treatment.

Male Pattern Baldness: The most common type of hair loss in men, which is characterized by hair loss at the crown and/ or a thinning or receding hair line.

Female Pattern Baldness: Hair loss that occurs in a uniform fashion across the scalp. In women, the crown may be affected. Yet, the hair loss rarely mimics the pattern of male pattern baldness.

Trichotillomania: A mental disorder that is characterized by the obsessive compulsive behavior of pulling out one's own hair. A person with this disorder will have noticeable missing patches of hair. The cause is unknown.

Psoriasis: An autoimmune disease that is characterized by red, silvery, scaly patches that can appear in the scalp as well as the rest of the body. This disease is treated with medication that can go directly on the scalp. Severe disease is also treated with oral medications.

Notes

Notes

_____

_____

_____

_____

_____

_____

_____

_____

_____

_____

_____

_____

_____

_____

_____

_____

Notes

_____

_____

_____

_____

_____

_____

_____

_____

_____

_____

_____

_____

_____

_____

_____

_____

_____

Notes

Transitioning

So—where are my ladies who have been chemically straightening your hair or getting a relaxer for many years who now wish to transition to natural hair but don't know where to start? Trust me, I know exactly how much anxiety you guys have because I was in your position years ago after I had a traumatic hair experience when I finished medical school.

I wanted to grow my relaxer out after taking out my sew-in extensions. I did not know how to style my hair, and I was too scared to cut off the relaxed portion of my hair. As a makeshift solution, I decided to rock sew-in extensions for several years because I did not want to relax my hair. Yet, I also did not want to display my natural hair because I did not know what to do with it. I know there is someone out there who will benefit from reading this chapter, and I wish you much success on your transition to healthy hair. Do not be afraid to embrace your own natural beauty. I wish I had embraced my natural hair much sooner than I did. Never doubt for one second that your hair is beautiful.

The first question you are most likely asking yourself is, should I "big chop" the relaxed portion of my hair or should I transition long-term? There is no correct answer to this question. It depends on the individual. I transitioned long-term because I had always had hair that was shoulder length or longer for most of my life. I couldn't see myself with a "struggle" fro . . . LOL! I held on to my hair until the new growth was so long that I no longer had anymore relaxed hair. I eventually had someone clip my ends before I had my extensions re-installed.

There is nothing wrong with transitioning long-term. However, you must keep in mind that your hair (especially the ends) will be very prone to dryness. You will definitely have a time managing your hair on wash days because you will have two to three hair textures to deal with as you progress with your transitioning process. An important part of your strands to focus on throughout the transitioning process is the line of demarcation (where your natural texture meets your relaxed texture). This portion of your strands is *the most fragile* point of your hair. If you do not choose to big chop your hair at the line of demarcation, then you have to be very careful with your hair throughout the long-term transitioning process. If you are the type of person who has trouble committing to a routine, then I would not recommend transitioning long-term. Instead, you can trim all your relaxed hair and enjoy your natural texture.

Can't decide whether to go for the big chop or a long-term transition? Don't worry—I got y'all. I have the top habits of successful transitioning for you.

1. **Cut off all the dead weight.** I know you love your hair, but you will be cutting the relaxed ends of your hair any-

way. Any damaged or split ends must go now. The longer you decide to transition will have a direct effect on the dryness and brittleness of the ends of your hair. This will help you prevent losing more hair later. Trust me!

2. **Pay close attention to the ends of your hair.** Like I just said, they will be dry and brittle. It is imperative that you prevent split ends. You will eventually be cutting them off completely. It might be a good idea to start trimming them regularly every four to six weeks depending on how fast your hair grows. And remember—please don't use your G-mama's old dull scissors to cut your hair yourself. Dull scissors cause split ends.

3. **Wash hair in sections.** You will have different textures of hair with the increased length of your new growth. Tangling will become an issue. Excessive tangling will promote breakage of your hair. You can decrease this by washing and detangling hair in four sections. This may not be necessary until you have been transitioning for at least three to four months.

4. **Pre-poo every time before you shampoo your hair.** If you haven't figured it out by now, your hair will be dry and prone to breakage. Your hair will need moisture, gentle detangling, and strengthening every week. I recommend you pre-poo for at least an hour before shampooing your hair.

5. **Be careful detangling your hair.** You should never attempt to detangle your hair without conditioners that contain lots of slip. You should always work in sections. Please don't try to comb through your hair with shampoo

in it. I can't stress enough how weak your hair will be at the line of demarcation.

6. **Deep condition your hair at least once per week.** Deep conditioning is a great way to restore the moisture–protein balance of your hair. Protein treatments or deep conditioners that contain protein are also a great way to replenish the hair cuticle.

7. **Limit or eliminate heat from your hair regimen as much as possible.** This is only going to cause damage to the healthy natural hair that you are trying to grow. It will also damage the ends, making them more prone to dryness, split ends, and subsequent breakage.

8. **Moisturize your hair like crazy.** Moisture will nourish your new growth and protect the ends of your hair to prevent split ends and breakage. You seemingly will never be able to moisturize your hair enough as you are transitioning from a relaxer to your natural curls/coils.

9. **Protective styles can help you transition.** You ladies also have the option to transition while using wigs, hair pieces, or weaves as a protective style while you transition. This is exactly what I did. You cannot neglect the hair that is growing underneath your extensions. You must still moisturize, deep condition, and trim your hair as needed. As a physician, I must remind you about traction alopecia from tight braids and hair pieces that tug at your hairline. The edges are a black woman's kryptonite. This is the most easily damaged part of your hair when wearing extensions. Don't lose your edges trying to be cute with these tight

sew-ins, U-parts, or wigs! I'm laughing, but I see this so often.

I do have a couple of secrets that will help you transitioning naturalistas through your hair struggles as you transition from a relaxer to your natural hair texture.

1. **Invest in head bands and head wraps.** They are great for covering your edges and pulling your hair back in a puff once you take down your twists or braids. Headbands can also cover up your unruly new growth and help smooth down your edges on a bad hair day.

2. **Avoid ponytails.** Ponytails put way too much stress on your hair at the line of demarcation and can lead to excessive breakage.

3. **Purchase a satin bonnet or satin pillowcase.** This will prevent you from drying out your hair on a cotton pillowcase. It will also help lengthen the life of your curly puffs, twist outs, or braid outs.

4. **Try to learn how to twist your hair, especially the flat twist.** Twisting your hair while wet and then removing the twists after allowing your hair to air dry is a great way to get your relaxed hair to mimic the texture of your natural hair. You're welcome!

Notes

Notes

Notes

Notes

Moisturizing Your Hair

All right, I hope you guys are still following me. This section is the most important part of the book. This information has taken me years and cost me thousands of dollars to figure out. Have you guys ever wondered how your best friend can use a product on her hair with amazing results just to have the exact opposite happen in your hair once you have attempted to use that very same product? I know your frustrations, and this chapter is here to help solve this problem. Why is it that the same product can be moisturizing for one naturalista but have horrendous results for the next? You have to factor in your hair texture and hair porosity along with the hair type. You must also try to use products on your hair by themselves before you start to cocktail them with other products.

One of the most popular methods to moisturize natural hair that you can easily find on any blog or YouTube video is the **LOC method**. The letters represent:

- Liquid (water or water-based leave-in conditioner)

- Cream moisturizer (or styling product)

- Oil

There are many variations to this method because of the expanding range of products that are available in the natural hair products industry. I cannot stress enough at this point how good just plain old water is for the hair as a moisturizer. I have been asked this countless times by many different women who want to make sure that wetting their hair every day is okay. You can wet your hair every day as long as you don't try to leave your house with dripping wet hair in the dead of winter. There are lots of great water-based leave-in conditioners. You can confirm that the leave-in you are already using is water-based by looking at the first three ingredients in the product. If one of the first three ingredients is not water, then the product is not water-based. There is also a noteworthy difference between a **penetrating oil** and a **sealing oil**. Examples of penetrating oil (which are named as such because it penetrates the hair shaft) are coconut oil, avocado oil, and olive oil. Examples of sealing oil (named as such because it seals the hair shaft) are castor oil, grapeseed oil, and jojoba oil. Penetrating oils should be used to infuse the hair cuticle with moisture while sealing oils should be used to prevent moisture loss by sealing the cuticle. If you are going to use a sealing oil in your hair regimen, then you should use the cream first or LCO method.

TESTS TO DETERMINE YOUR HAIR POROSITY

I have to be honest with you guys. I determined my porosity solely by how it responded to hair products. I was experimenting with so many different products as I scoured the Internet and YouTube for information to supplement my curiosity about my natural 3b and 3c curls. I did come across a test on YouTube called the **strand test**. You must take one of your clean, dry hair strands and place it in a glass of water. High-porosity hair sinks almost immediately while low-porosity hair floats indefinitely on the water. Normal-porosity hair will start to sink eventually, albeit not as fast, as high-porosity hair. If you are really curious about the results, this test should be easy to perform at home.

TIPS FOR MOISTURIZING LOW-POROSITY HAIR

(Your main objective should be to get your hair to absorb more water or water-based moisturizers.)

1. **Pay close attention to your hair's product buildup.** I know, I know—I am not the biggest fan of shampooing my hair. For the folks with low-porosity hair, you may have to use a shampoo a bit more frequently than I do because products tend to build up faster on your hair. This will make moisturizing you hair virtually impossible if you are trying to moisturize your hair in the face of excess product buildup.

2. **Invest in a steamer to steam your hair.** Heat opens up the

hair cuticle. This is a great option before moisturizing your hair after clarifying and washing it. You can also use the steam when applying your deep conditioning treatment.

3. **Deep condition your hair with heat.** If you can't afford a hooded hair dryer or a steamer, you can always get plastic caps or old plastic grocery bags to cover your hair to use your body heat. Plastic caps and head wraps are great options if you work out a lot or have to cover your hair at work.

4. **Learn what products have an acidic or basic pH.** You will need to use a product with an alkaline (basic) pH to open the cuticle of your hair strands and a different leave-in conditioner with an acidic pH to close your hair cuticle. Once you figure out what products to use, this will elevate your hair game with the quickness.

TIPS FOR MOISTURIZING NORMAL TO HIGH-POROSITY HAIR

(Your main objective should be infusing moisture and restoring the protein composition of your hair strands.)

1. **Apple Cider Vinegar (ACV):** This substance is beneficial for treating dandruff and hair loss, removing product buildup, and restoring hair/scalp pH. This is a substance with acidic properties that can decrease the porosity of your hair. I have seen ACV in several different deep conditioning masks for high-porosity naturalistas.

2. **Aloe Vera:** One of the miracle ingredients that will infuse moisture to your strands. It doesn't matter if you use aloe vera juice or aloe vera gel. Your high-porosity hair will love it. You can thank me later.

3. **Deep Conditioning:** Deep conditioning treatments are a great way to restore your protein.

4. **Coconut Oil:** Coconut oil is a penetrating oil that is known for restoring moisture and protein to hair strands, which makes it a high-porosity hair diva's best friend.

Now, as much as I have been preaching about moisturizing your hair to you guys, I don't want you to think that you cannot overdo it. Have you guys ever heard the saying that alludes to too much of a good thing becoming bad for you? Well, this is the sentiment with moisture. Low elasticity is one of the main indicators that you may be over moisturizing your hair. If you have noticed that when you stretch your hair while it's wet that it does not return to its normal state, then you most likely have low elasticity.

The key to restoring the elasticity in your strands is to find the perfect balance between moisture and protein in your strands. Hair that has been treated with too much protein is characteristically dry, stiff, and brittle. Excessive protein treatments can cause your strands to experience a phenomenon known as **protein sensitivity** or **protein overload**. Overly moisturized hair tends to feel very "mushy" and limp due to the low elasticity and is a strong indication that you may need to use a protein treatment to rebuild the protein structure of your hair. This phenomenon of mushy hair is known as moisture overload or hygral fatigue. **Moisture overload** or **hygral fatigue** is the result of the constant swelling of the hair cuticle as moisture is absorbed and the contraction of the hair cuticle as it dries. Hygral fatigue exposes your strands to stress via excessive stretching, and ultimately leads to breakage.

Habits that lead to hygral fatigue are:

1. Deep conditioning longer than recommended times by manufacturer

2. Exclusive use of deep conditioning treatment that has no protein

3. Excessively wetting the hair without letting it dry completely

4. Incessant overnight conditioning of your curls on wash days

If you believe your strands are suffering from hygral fatigue, then you should consider these preventative measures to help your strands recover:

1. Pre-poo with olive oil, coconut oil, or avocado oil to reduce the amount of swelling of your cuticles on wash days. These oils are penetrating oils that can penetrate the hair shaft.

2. Limit the amount of time that you drench your hair in water. That means you need to stop deep conditioning your hair overnight.

3. Close the cuticle by using pH-balanced products.

Notes

_____

_____

_____

_____

_____

_____

_____

_____

_____

_____

_____

_____

_____

_____

_____

_____

_____

Notes

Notes

Notes

Shrinkage

I know some of you guys are thinking that you have been doing all of the things we have discussed thus far—*but* your healthy, moisturized hair never falls below your shoulders when in its natural state. When blown out, your hair may reach your bra strap. This short length of your hair in its natural curly state is most likely due to the shrinkage of your type 3 or type 4 curls. Shrinkage is the difference in the length of your hair when stretched to its maximum length (blown out or straightened) versus when your strands are washed and conditioned, then allowed to dry in its natural state. Shrinkage can affect all curls from type 2 to type 4, but it is especially noticeable in type 4 curls because they tend to be the tightest. I have seen some #Curlfriends lose as much as eight inches to shrinkage once their hair dries.

Most of my #Curlfriends probably want to avoid shrinkage like the plague because they want to appreciate some of the styling benefits of having longer tresses. Fighting shrinkage can be very damaging to your strands if you are stretching or applying excessive amounts of heat to the hair and scalp. Let's discuss how to minimize the shrinkage in your hair. We have already mentioned the **blow out**, which is simply blow drying your hair. You must be careful with the heat settings on your blow dryer, but this is a great option if you have long hair and want to wear your hair in a soft-braided updo or trim your ends.

There are several heat-free alternatives to the blow out that will minimize the shrinkage of your curls:

1. **Banding:** Banding is the process of gently stretching wet, moisturized hair using ponytail holders. It is imperative that ouchless (no metal clasp) ponytail holders are used to decrease breakage. The ponytail holder is wrapped around the length of your strands from root to tip after parting the hair into one of many sections.

2. **African Threading:** This is pretty much the same process as banding, but thread is used instead of ouchless ponytail holders. A special technique is used to wrap the thread around individual sections of hair to stretch it while it is drying as in banding.

3. **Bantu Knots:** Bantu knots are not "knots." They are actually sections of hair, coiled or wound into a small bun with the ends pinned or tucked underneath the bun. This elongates your tight coils into voluminous and looser bouncy curls.

4. **Sets:** There are multiple options available to "set" the hair like flexi-rods, straw rollers, curl formers, rollers, etc. Usually, the hair is set while wet after washing and conditioning. After the hair is set, the individual must sit under a hooded dryer to dry the hair.

5. Twists and Braids: Two-strand twists and braids are an easy way to elongate the hair and also allow you to see your true length when your hair is sectioned into two to four twists or braids on wash day. Braids create more stretch or tension than twists and will give your strands a little extra length.

Shrinkage is not the worst thing in the world for you, #Curlfriends. In fact, shrinkage indicates that your strands have optimal health. An increased amount of shrinkage in curly/coily hair indicates that your hair has a great amount of elasticity. Remember in a previous chapter where elasticity was discussed? Well, strands that lack elasticity are more prone to breakage. Any chemical or physical process such as relaxers or excessive heat "relaxes" the curl of your strands so much that it can lead to a loss of elasticity and subsequent breakage.

Did you know that hair that shrinks is actually more versatile and fun than hair that isn't? You can have a curly/coily puff or afro on one day, straighten your hair on another day, and maybe have a messy bun or twist out on another day. You can have several different hairstyles in the course of just one week. Women who do not have textured hair like my #Curlfriends can't have the fun that we have with our hair. This most likely explains why some women who do not have this type of hair always want to try to touch your hair at school and work. You can express yourself and your personality through many unique hairstyles. This is one of the great benefits of shrinkage.

There is no way for us to get away from shrinkage. However, we need to embrace our shrinkage, #Curlfriends.

Shrinkage is one of those things that makes our hair what it is. I totally get that you guys may be frustrated that people cannot see the true length of your beautiful hair. Yet, you guys should definitely not forget about the health of your strands. I know sometimes your hair may be a tangly mess of single strand knots or prone to dryness and breakage at times, but embracing your natural texture means that you can be unapologetically you with versatile, fun, and cute natural hair (with a little or a lot of shrinkage).

Notes

_____

_____

_____

_____

_____

_____

_____

_____

_____

_____

_____

_____

_____

_____

_____

_____

_____

Notes

Notes

_____

_____

_____

_____

_____

_____

_____

_____

_____

_____

_____

_____

_____

_____

_____

_____

_____

_____

_____

Notes

Hair Growth and Length Retention

A popular misconception that many of you reading this book may have is that your hair "doesn't grow." Your hair is growing at a steady rate *all the time*. The cells that are dividing in the hair bulb eventually push out of the scalp and are covered with a layer of keratin once they become part of the hair shaft. The problem is not at the roots of your hair. It is on the ends of your hair! Remember when I mentioned that the ends are the oldest part of your hair? Well, the ends of your hair serve as the source of the length retention problem that many of you may have. It is also imperative that you ladies do not confuse alopecia with traumatic breakage or damage. There is no cause for alopecia, but there is a cause for traumatic damage/breakage.

Here are some other common reasons why you may not have noticeable hair growth:

1. **Shrinkage** causes hair to appear much shorter than it is when blown out or straightened.
2. **Dry and brittle hair** leads to breakage.

3. **Not loving the ends of your hair** leads to breakage and split ends.

4. **Using inappropriate or ineffective styling tools** leads to breakage and split ends.

5. **Genetics** lead to hair loss and is sometimes unavoidable and uncontrollable.

6. **Poor diet** leads to unwanted hair loss.

7. **Hair trauma** can be from chemical process or poor care.

8. **Health issues/medications** lead to unwanted hair loss.

MOST COMMON MEDICAL CONDITIONS THAT CAUSE HAIR LOSS:

Iron deficiency/anemia: When your blood levels of iron (Fe) or hemoglobin are too low, you can become anemic and lose hair as a result. Normal levels of vitamin B are also critical to maintaining healthy hair.

Hyper/hypothyroid disease: Thyroid disease occurs when the normal production of thyroid hormones, triiodothyronine (T3) and thyroxine (T4), are disrupted. Thyroid hormones contribute to such a wide range of processes throughout the body that impaired thyroid function can stall hair growth. Hair loss is a common side effect of many medications. Most of the time, these drugs only cause temporary hair loss that goes away once you've adjusted to or stopped taking the medicine. These medications damage the hair follicles themselves, disrupting growth at different stages.

COMMON MEDICATIONS THAT CAUSE HAIR LOSS:

Vitamin A: High doses of vitamin A and medications derived from it can cause hair loss.

Acne medications: Two types of vitamin A-derived acne medication, isotretinoin (Accutane) and tretinoin (Retin-A) can cause hair loss. You may want to discuss other options with your dermatologist or primary doctor because this drug has several other serious side effects besides hair loss.

Antibiotics: Prescription antibiotics can cause temporary hair thinning by depleting your vitamin B and hemoglobin, which disrupts hair growth. As discussed earlier, normal levels of vitamin B and iron are also critical to maintaining healthy hair.

Antifungals: An antifungal medication, voriconazole, is one such treatment that has been associated with alopecia in the past.

Anti-clotting drugs: Anticoagulants like heparin and warfarin are used to thin the blood and prevent blood clots and certain health concerns in some people (like those with heart conditions). These medications can cause hair loss that begins after taking these medications for about three months.

Cholesterol-lowering drugs: Some statin drugs like simvastatin (Zocor) and atorvastatin (Lipitor) have been reported to cause hair loss.

Immunosuppressants: Some immune-suppressing drugs used to treat autoimmune conditions like lupus and rheumatoid arthritis can cause hair loss. A few of these include methotrexate, leflunomide (Arava), cyclophosphamide (Cytoxan), and etanercept (Enbrel).

Anticonvulsants: Medications that prevent seizures, like valproic acid (Depakote) and trimethadione (Tridione), can lead to hair loss in some people.

Blood pressure medications: Medications that are used to help control the blood pressure can lead to hair loss. Beta-blockers act on the beta-adrenergic receptors of the cardiovascular system and cause the heart to beat more slowly when taken.

Beta-blockers, including the following, can cause hair loss:
- metoprolol (Lopressor)
- timolol (Blocadren)
- propranolol (Inderal and Inderal LA)
- atenolol (Tenormin)
- nadolol (Corgard)

ACE inhibitors can also lead to thinning hair. ACE inhibitors inhibit the production of angiotensin II in the body, which lowers the blood pressure by causing your blood vessels to dilate. The ACE inhibitors that lead to hair loss include:

- enalapril (Vasotec)

- lisinopril (Prinivil, Zestril)

- captopril (Capoten)

Antidepressants and mood stabilizers: Some people who take medications for depression and mood stabilization may also experience hair loss.

Drugs that may cause this include:

- paroxetine hydrochloride (Paxil)

- sertraline (Zoloft)

- protriptyline (Vivactil)

- amitriptyline (Elavil)

- fluoxetine (Prozac)

Weight loss drugs: Weight loss medications like phentermine can cause hair loss, but the side effect isn't often listed. This is because dieters who lose their hair are often also nutrient-deficient or may have underlying health conditions contributing to their hair loss. In these instances, hair loss may be due to poor nutrition instead of the weight loss medication.

Medications for gout: Gout medications like allopurinol (Zyloprim and Lopurin) have been reported to cause hair loss.

Chemotherapy: Chemotherapy drugs used to treat certain types of cancer and autoimmune illness can cause anagen effluvium. This hair loss includes eyelashes, eyebrows, and body hair.

These drugs are designed to destroy the fast-growing cancer cells in your body, but they also attack and destroy other cells that grow quickly, like the roots of your hair. Regrowth will occur after treatments have ended.

As you can see, there are more than a few medications that can keep your hair from growing or cause it to appear very thin and fragile. I know it is challenging to stay on top of your medical issues and maintain the length and thickness that you desire for your hair. In some instances, stopping the medication may not be an option. I would encourage anyone taking any of these medications that were listed to have a conversation with their healthcare professional about what should be done to maintain your hair while taking these medications.

For the past year or so, I have been retaining more length in my natural hair because I have changed my hair regimen to support length retention and stimulate healthy growth. One of the most effective changes I made was to stop straightening my hair with heat. I was noticing that my curl pattern had started to become nonexistent after continually using a flat iron to straighten my hair to blend my natural hair with some textured clip-ins that I purchased on Black Friday in 2016. My hair had become weak, dry, and brittle, and my curls were not as healthy looking as they were in December 2016. I decided that I was not going to let this situation defeat me.

I quit the clip-ins cold turkey in June 2017 and stopped straightening my hair. I started using natural hair products to enhance my natural curl pattern and repair the damage that had been done to my hair for the past six months. I actually cut off the damaged portion because I knew there was no saving it. I knew enough about damaged ends stunting the growth of healthy hair to come to terms with the fact that my damaged ends had to go. I began deep conditioning my hair and moisturizing it on a regular basis. I stopped applying heat to my hair as well. I also started taking biotin, iron, and vitamin C supplements. As a result, I have retained six inches of growth in the past twelve months.

What can you do to retain length if your hair is suffering from heat and chemical damage? You can definitely learn from the mistakes I made when I damaged my own hair almost two years ago. First, you need to take an honest assessment of your own hair. You must ask yourself what parts of your hair are damaged and how this damage occurred. If you are unsure, please consult a licensed professional. Once you have assessed the damage, please do not try to save brittle, dry, lifeless split ends that are hanging on for dear life. Also, if you have been using heat on your hair to straighten it, please invest in a good heat protectant. A good heat protectant is the one essential step that I was missing when I was using heat on my hair. One caution is that heat protectants often contain silicone-derived ingredients that coat the hair and lead to buildup if not washed out properly. Do not use your flat iron on your hair every day (like I did). Finally, you must develop a regimen where you clarify your hair regularly to remove product buildup, use protein treatments every four to six weeks, and deep condition your hair at least once a week. After three months, reassess the damaged portions of your hair and trim any portion that is still damaged.

In summary . . .

ROUTINE TO REJUVENATE HEAT/CHEMICAL DAMAGED HAIR:

1. **Assess damage.** You must perform an initial trim if hair is severely damaged.

2. **Limit heat.** If you must straighten your hair during this time, please use a heat protectant. Also, please refrain from excessive flat iron use after your hair is straightened.

3. **Clarify your hair.** This prevents product buildup and will help your hair absorb the protein and deep conditioning treatments that will help rejuvenate your tired tresses.

4. **Use a protein treatment and/or deep conditioners with protein/amino acids in them.** Protein will help rebuild the damaged portions of your cuticle and restore your curls.

5. **Reassess the damage at three months.** Trim damaged ends again if necessary.

At this point, I know the next question some of you have is, how can I treat hair loss or alopecia?

There are two types of alopecia, scarring and non-scarring. **Scarring alopecia** normally leads to irreversible hair loss. **Non-scarring alopecia** is treated with various penetrating hair oils that penetrate the hair follicle in the scalp and the hair shaft. Castor oil is the most widely used penetrating oil used to help regain your hair loss from non-scarring alopecia. Sometimes castor oil loses its effectiveness. In these cases, it is beneficial to look into other acceptable alternatives such as rosemary, ylang ylang, and sage oils. Some combination of these oils is put into most stimulating scalp oils and serums in the market currently that aid in healthy scalp and hair growth. The oil or serum is dropped onto the scalp in sections where the individual is experiencing alopecia and then rubbed into the scalp. Scalp massages also help the oils penetrate the scalp and stimulate the hair follicle.

If you are really committed to retaining more length in your strands, then you should focus on healthy moisturized strands and a healthy scalp. You may want to keep a hair journal to keep track of the products and ingredients that cause your strands to flourish. Don't get caught up in measuring your hair because your curls/coils will display a fair amount of shrinkage if they have adequate elasticity. If you have a solid hair regimen with little to no breakage or damage, keep doing what you are doing. If you have begun to notice that your alopecia is not resolving after months of treatment, please see a medical professional to rule out scarring alopecia.

Notes

Notes

_____

_____

_____

_____

_____

_____

_____

_____

_____

_____

_____

_____

_____

_____

_____

_____

_____

_____

Notes

Notes

_____

_____

_____

_____

_____

_____

_____

_____

_____

_____

_____

_____

_____

_____

_____

_____

_____

_____

Protective Styling

So now you are noticing that your hair is growing with sustainable length retention and you want to know if protective styles can help you maintain your overall hair health and protect your hair from split ends and breakage—right? Well this is the main reason that most women use protective styles, regardless if they are natural or relaxed. A protective style is any style where the ends of your hair are tucked away. Remember that your ends are the oldest and most fragile part of your hair, so they need constant love and attention. A protective style also protects your hair from other external factors that result in damage and breakage. These hairstyles include braids, twists, updos, wigs, and weaves, which can also add another fun way to express your personality through your hair without damaging it.

Why do most naturalistas use protective styling in their hair? The most common reason that I have encountered is to give themselves a break. Dealing with your natural hair can be hard work, especially if you have a lot of hair. Some protective styles are installed to help improve the overall health of an individual's hair. An example of this phenomenon is still being able to clean, condition, and moisturize the hair while it's in a low-manipulation protective style. Finally, another good reason to install a protective style is to prevent breakage. If you have been noticing that your hair is dry and frizzy, it may be a good idea to install a protective style to give your hair some extra time to repair while continuing your healthy hair regimen.

A popular way to protect your tresses from the stress and increased manipulation of daily styling is to wear a wig. Wigs are a great way to try different hairstyles and hair colors without exposing your hair to any damaging heat or chemicals. However, you cannot neglect your own hair underneath your wigs. You must continue a healthy hair regimen.

Here are my top tips for healthy wig wearing:

1. **Watch your edges.** That means choosing a wig that fits your head properly and with nylon netting that lets your scalp and hairline breathe. You also need to watch the tension on combs or hairpins that are used to secure the wig. These can cause tension alopecia. Gel wig liners can protect your hairline and your skin.

2. **Please don't take care of your wigs better than your own hair underneath the wig.** This means you must shampoo, condition, deep condition, and moisturize your hair and scalp underneath the wig. You will defeat the purpose of wearing a wig as a protective style if you neglect your own hair. If you are a person who sweats a lot or wears her wig while working out, please make sure to wash your hair and the wig unit, please.

3. **Don't put the wig on wet or damp hair.** This will provide a breeding ground for germs and fungus. Damp hair can also cause your wig unit to mildew. Mildew causes the wig to smell terribly. Trust me—this is not the look or smell you want if you are trying to be fly.

4. **Scalp massages and wig breaks are your friend.** You want to give your scalp and hair some time to breathe and get some vitamin D or sunlight. It will also give you time to wash and care for your hair properly so it continues to grow healthy and strong.

5. **Avoid bunching your hair up underneath a wig cap.** Keeping your hair balled up under a wig cap can lead to hair breakage and damage. Braids that lie flat on your scalp or cornrows are a great option to protect your hair while wearing your wig unit. Cornrows will also help the wig lie flat on your head.

Sew-ins and weaves are popular protective styles for my #Curl-friends who may be transitioning from relaxed to natural hair. Weaves can be a protective style gone bad if special attention is not given to the maintenance of the weave and your own natural hair throughout the duration of your install.

My top tips for protecting your hair while wearing a weave or extensions:

1. **Please get your weave installed by a licensed profession-al**. I can't tell you how many times I have seen a woman with poorly and very tightly installed hair extensions that were damaging her edges so badly that I could tell by taking a glancing at her. A professional will also be able to

let you know how often you should have follow-up hair appointments for proper weave maintenance. Having a professional help you with weave maintenance will also make most of my other tips easier for you.

2. **Make sure your weave is not sewn in or braided too tightly at your hairline.** I said it before, and I'll say it again. Edges are the black woman's kryptonite, the weakest part of your hair. They are not meant to be snatched by tight-fitting hairpieces or braids. You can cause so much inflammation of the hair follicle that your traction alopecia will become permanent hair loss. I am on a quest to save as many women's edges as I can, so please listen when I say to watch how tight your installation braids are underneath your sew-in and watch how tightly sewn your tracks are to your hairline.

3. **Shampoo, condition, and style your weave on a regular basis.** This is a very important step in weave maintenance to prevent fungus or mold growing inside your weave. You must make sure you dry your braids and weave completely when washing because damp, dark environments support the growth of organisms such as fungus and mold. It smells terrible and will cause hair loss.

4. **Moisturize your own hair that is underneath your extensions.** It is definitely a good idea to oil your scalp with a light oil like almond oil or jojoba oil to decrease the chance of clogged pores and product buildup. If you want to clarify your braided hair underneath your installation, an apple cider vinegar rinse may be just the thing you need to help with cleaning your hair and scalp.

5. Consider supplementing your routine with a hair vitamin. A hair vitamin supplement will help to ensure that your growing hair will be strong and healthy. It will help your hair continue to grow after you have removed your protective style.

Braids and twists are a common protective style used to promote length retention and decrease breakage in your hair when they are installed and cared for properly.

My top tips for you hair divas who are fans of braided styles are:

1. Again . . . watch those edges. Please! If you already have thin and sensitive edges, please know that you are at a higher risk of traction alopecia than others. This is why you should keep the braids loose, especially at your hairline. I have seen too many women with no edges after getting Senegalese twists or other small braids that damaged their hairlines severely. Remember that this is the black woman's kryptonite!

2. Wearing your braids for longer than four to six weeks without touch-ups can damage your hair. You will need to touch up your braids, especially at the hairline. If you do not, this can result in breakage or traction alopecia.

3. Smaller braids can cause your hair to become thin. I know that micro braids are beautiful, but please remember that repetitive installation of micro braids can thin your hair over time and cause decreased length retention. Having thin hair is a quick way to have the opposite desired effects from a protective style.

4. **Braids will help with length retention, but they do not "make your hair grow."** Braids are considered a low manipulation style because your ends are braided together in several braids. However, your hair is at risk of damage and breakage every time you detangle and style your hair. You decrease your chances of breakage and increase length retention with braided hairstyles. Just choose braided styles wisely and refresh your braids as needed while still caring for your hair properly.

Notes

Notes

Notes

Notes

Natural Hair Product Ingredients

Have you ever been in the store with the intention to buy some hair products to whip your hair in shape, only to look on the back of the container to realize that you don't know what half of the ingredients are? Well, this chapter is for you. I am going to break down ingredients that you want to see in your products, ingredients that are known hazards, and some of the ingredients you may want to avoid based on your hair type or overall health.

There has been an increasing amount of alarming news reports that indicate dangerous chemicals called endocrine disruptors are being used in hair products that are marketed to black women. With this disturbing information and the ever-growing list of brands in the market, choosing hair products to supplement each part of your hair regimen can be a daunting task. I have tried to simplify this process by discussing ingredients by their product category. I hope this information empowers my #Curlfriends to buy products that help maintain optimal hair health and keep their curls/coils looking their best without sacrificing their health.

Zakiya Antoine, DO, MPH

Have you ever looked at the labels of your favorite natural hair brands and wondered why most of them have labels that refute the presence of propylene glycol, parabens, pthalates, mineral oils, paraffin, synthetic fragrance, or synthetic color? Well, there is definitely a reason why you should be concerned about these ingredients. This brings me back to that term, endocrine disruptors, which I mentioned earlier.

Endocrine disruptors are chemicals that compete with hormone receptors in the human body. These chemicals can then hinder, mimic, or augment the response of this particular hormone in the human body. It is believed this may correlate to black women having a higher incidence of uterine fibroids, infertility, and other female reproductive issues. **Parabens** have been widely used as broad-spectrum preservatives in hair products and are known endocrine disruptors that have been linked to breast cancer since 2005. More extensive scientific research needs to be conducted for causality and correlation. Since the original study that linked antiperspirant use to breast tumors, many cosmetic companies have halted the use of parabens in their formulations of their products in the market. Similarly, pthalates have been suggested to disrupt the function of estrogen in breast tissue and have been linked to breast cancer.

Pthalates were commonly used as emulsifiers, which help ingredients in hair products mix together.

Propylene glycol is used as a surfactant (cleansing agent), humectant (moisturizing agent), or emulsifier in hair products, but they are causing lots of controversy due to the risk of allergic reaction that can result in skin rashes or asthma exacerbation. Mineral oil, paraffin, or other crude oil derivatives are controversial ingredients because of the filtering process that must occur when these substances are separated from crude oil. There is a concern that all cancerous/harmful chemicals are not removed from some of these oils while in their filtration process. Most natural hair products will not ever use mineral oils. Finally, synthetic colors and fragrances are avoided because they are not regulated by the FDA, and it is unknown how much of a potentially toxic substance may be used in the formulation of the fragrance or color. If you notice that synthetic fragrance is one of the last ingredients on the packaging, it may be safe to assume that there is not much of a risk because there is very little of the fragrance/ color in the formulation of the product.

When considering the ingredients of products that can clarify and cleanse your hair, I want my #Curlfriends to remember the substances that should be avoided, the substances that should be used with caution, and the substances that are widely used in shampoos or co-washes. You guys already know that the substances to avoid are parabens and pthalates, but there is an ingredient that should be approached with caution: **sulfates**. Sulfates are cleansing agents that cause shampoos to lather. Most of my #Curlfriends may want to steer clear of sulfates because they can lead to dryness and subsequent damage of your hair; and they can strip the color from color-treated hair. Sulfate-containing shampoos can also lead to dry scalp. If you work out or swim frequently,

I would avoid sulfate-containing shampoos altogether. Sulfate-containing shampoos are considered clarifying shampoos, and they are used by some with naturally curly hair that use silicone-containing products to moisturize or condition their hair. It is thought you need to strip the silicone film from your hair to ensure there is little or no product buildup in your hair. This brings me back to an earlier point I made about using sulfate-free shampoos or co-washes to clarify your hair. This also explains the need to do a pre-poo treatment before using any type of shampoo on your hair. Sulfate-free shampoos are widely used in the natural hair care industry. I personally use sulfate-free shampoos at least one to two times per month.

Moisturizing your hair is one of the most important steps in a healthy hair regimen. It can be very confusing when products that are supposed to moisturize your hair contain ingredients that can hinder optimal moisture levels or may be harmful to your health. As previously stated several times, most well-known controversial and potentially harmful ingredients are not in the formulation of natural hair products. The main ingredients you need to be cautious of are synthetic fragrances, propylene glycols, and silicones. Propylene glycol is known for being a good humectant. Caution is advised with propylene glycol because of a possible allergic reaction to these products. There are no known toxicities, but many women complain of rashes or asthma exacerbation after exposure to this chemical, which is why many companies avoid this substance in their formulations.

Synthetic fragrance has been linked to allergic reactions and potential for toxicity/carcinogenicity because it is currently not regulated by the FDA. Silicones coat your strands and are substances that are added to leave-in conditioners to add shine, add slip to the products to help with detangling, and also decrease frizz in humid conditions. Silicones even offer the benefits of heat and color protection due to the sealing and protective layer they add to your strands. It is this same layer of protection that causes their controversy. Many argue that you must clarify your hair with a sulfate-containing shampoo once per month if you use products with silicones because silicones can cause product buildup in your hair. These shampoos can cause many problems with stripping the color and moisture from your hair while also causing damage, as discussed earlier in this chapter. However, you can use water-soluble silicones that can be easily washed out with a co-wash or sulfate-free shampoo. It has been my experience to get my hair completely free of buildup if I just wash my hair twice with the sulfate-free shampoo (when I think it's necessary).

Deep conditioning treatments contain very few harmful ingredients. When choosing a deep conditioner, a fun but important fact to consider is the order of the ingredients on the packaging. The ingredients that are listed first are present in the highest concentrations in the actual product. This means that the ingredients falling last on the list are lower in concentration in the product. One of the first ingredients of your deep conditioner should be water (surprise). If one of the first three ingredients is not water, please don't purchase this product to treat your hair. Other common ingredients in deep conditioners are oils, Shea butter, and vegetable glycerin. These ingredients will aid with moisture and serve as a mixing medium for other ingredients and nutrients that are infused into deep conditioners. Protein and silicone are two ingredients that I want to caution my #Curlfriends to monitor carefully in these products. Protein is not dangerous but must not be used without proper knowledge of how often you should apply protein treatments to your hair. Silicones add great slip to your strands during application of the deep conditioner, but they can also lead to product buildup if not properly removed when clarifying the hair.

Natural styling products contain very few harmful ingredients that will cause worry for any of my #Curlfriends. Some common ingredients are water, aloe vera, horsetail, nettle, vitamin E, and essential oil blends. These products are great for adding some texture, hold, and volume to any hairstyle you want. I love applying my stylers to wet hair to decrease frizz and add volume to my curls. These products avoid all dangerous ingredients, but some styling products do contain silicones. As long as you have a good sulfate-free shampoo in your regimen, you should have little to no reservation about using any styling or twisting gel/cream.

Notes

Notes

Notes

_____

_____

_____

_____

_____

_____

_____

_____

_____

_____

_____

_____

_____

_____

_____

_____

_____

Notes

Natural Hair Care for Kids

All this buzz in the media about dangerous ingredients in black hair products is enough to make anyone give all products the side-eye before allowing them to be used in your hair and the hair of your babies. Black hair products are not the only products in the market that have been scrutinized for dangerous ingredients. In 2011, a popular baby brand's baby shampoo and baby wash were found to contain two ingredients, dioxane and quaternium-15, that were considered "harmful to babies." Considered a carcinogen, 1,4-Dioxane is used to make chemicals more soluble and gentler on the skin in these products, while quaternium-15 is a chemical preservative that kills bacteria by releasing formaldehyde (also a known carcinogen found in embalming fluid). Protecting our children from threats that are known and unknown is the number one priority for their parents. You should definitely stick to baby brands that disclose all ingredients in their products and strive to use as many natural and organic ingredients as possible. Popular baby brands definitely have a responsibility to make sure that they are not selling products with dangerous ingredients to the consumers who may be tempted to purchase their products.

The most helpful and important action you can take with your child's natural hair is to develop a routine as soon as possible, especially with a child who has a lot of hair. Children can be very temperamental and act up when it's "hair time." Just like meal time and bath time, your child should recognize that caring for their hair is a normal part of their day. Little girls (and boys with lots of hair) will need to develop patience when it's washday or time to refresh their hairstyle before they go to bed. You can do things to make this fun and set an example for your child by doing some steps in the routine together at bedtime. Your child will feel loved and cared for, especially if you tend to be busy and unavailable earlier in the day.

Another important lesson for you to teach your young ones is that their gorgeous curls/coils must be moisturized to keep it healthy and strong. The regimen that you should be using in your child's hair should include a natural, moisturizing leave-in conditioner and sealing the ends with oil. Leave-in conditioner is an important aid in detangling your child's curly/coily strands. You should never attempt to detangle your baby's hair without a leave-in moisturizing product in it. When you try to detangle dry hair, you will most likely struggle with an upset child who says you are hurting him or her and subsequently have damaging and messy results. Trust me—leave-in conditioner is your friend. You can use an oil as a sealant on the ends after you are done detangling your baby's hair.

With all of the problems with dryness and tangled hair, I know some of you are wondering whether it's okay to co-wash you child's hair. The answer to this question is yes. It may be necessary to rinse your child or toddler's hair daily if he or she tends to get food or other undesirable substances in his or her hair on a daily basis. A co-wash is a good way to clean your child's hair without causing it to be overly dry. You can use your favorite natural/organic baby brand conditioner to freshen your baby's soiled curls/coils in between shampoos.

Styling your child's hair can be an arduous task if you are using the wrong products. The "wrong" products are most likely drying your little one's hair to the point that it's hard for you to manipulate their hair while styling it. Products that dry the hair out also make it hard for your child's hairstyle to last past one to two days after going through the whole "process" to get your baby's hair looking presentable. Stylers that are acceptable to use in your little one's hair are created by natural and organic children's product lines and are usually called hair smoothies, gel moisturizers, or curling/defining custards. These are acceptable products to use in your children's hair to make it more manageable while styling. They can also aid in detangling the hair as well. You may want to invest in some barrettes or bows for your baby girl's hair.

Notes

Notes

_____

_____

_____

_____

_____

_____

_____

_____

_____

_____

_____

_____

_____

_____

_____

_____

Notes

Notes

Thank You

Thank you, #Curlfriends, from the bottom of my heart for purchasing and reading this book. This is my first book in my Strandtastic book series, and I would love your feedback and suggestions for things you would like to see in the next book. Don't be scared—I can take it. I hope that I have taught you a few things that you may not have realized about your naturally curly hair. Our natural hair is beautiful, isn't it?

You guys know that Dr. Zakiya is super busy! I'm either seeing a patient at a new locums assignment, on the tradeshow circuit speaking about or selling my natural hair products, or in the lab creating awesome new hair products. Soon, Dr. Zakiya may even be in a city near you as I travel the country to take care of my #Curlfriends who need specialized attention. Let's stay connected so I can keep you updated on my activities. Here's how:

Website: www.DrZakiyaAntoine.com

Facebook: www.facebook.com/DrZakiyaAntoine

Twitter: www.twitter.com/DrZakiyaAntoine

YouTube: www.youtube.com/user/DrZakiyaAntoine

Instagram: www.instagram.com/DrZakiyaAntoine

Pinterest: www.pinterest.com/DrZakiyaAntoine

LinkedIn: www.linkedin.com/in/DrZakiyaAntoine

About the Author

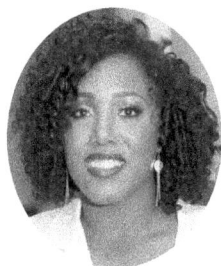

One of the nation's most acclaimed beauty experts and physicians, Zakiya Antoine, DO, MPH, is a board-certified family medicine physician, a nationally recognized author, speaker, health and wellness expert, and beauty brand CEO.

Known as the "Natural Hair Doctor," Dr. Zakiya travels the country instructing and providing healthcare to those in need. As the founder and chief medical advisor of DrZakiyaAntoine.com, she discusses actionable ideas and real-world strategies to help women take control of their health. Dr. Zakiya also shares medical expertise via her popular FB Live series to help her #Curlfriends pursue a healthier life. Her mission is simple: real medical advice, simplified.

Dr. Zakiya obtained a master of public health with a focus in epidemiology from Tulane University School of Public Health and Tropical Medicine, earned her doctor of osteopathic medicine from The Ohio University, completed her internship at University Hospitals of Cleveland System, and finished her family medicine residency at Michigan State University.

To learn more, visit her website at
www.DrZakiyaAntoine.com

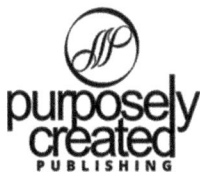

CREATING DISTINCTIVE BOOKS
WITH INTENTIONAL RESULTS

We're a collaborative group of creative masterminds with a mission to produce high-quality books to position you for monumental success in the marketplace.

Our professional team of writers, editors, designers, and marketing strategists work closely together to ensure that every detail of your book is a clear representation of the message in your writing.

Want to know more?
Write to us at info@publishyourgift.com
or call (888) 949-6228

Discover great books, exclusive offers, and more at
www.PublishYourGift.com

Connect with us on social media

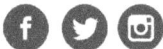

@publishyourgift